What Makes Your Heart Sing?

A GUIDE TO CREATING THEMES FOR YOGA CLASSES

By Noelle Cormier, ERYT

Produced by:

FriesenPress
Suite 300 – 852 Fort Street
Victoria, BC, Canada V8W 1H8

www.friesenpress.com

Distributed to the trade by The Ingram Book Company

Table of Contents

How to Use this Book

This book is intended for use in conjunction with a Certified Yoga Teacher Training Program. The information in this book is designed to provide information on the subjects discussed. The routines suggested are for educational purposes only and should not be attempted without the skillful guidance of a Certified Yoga Instructor. This book is not to be used, nor should it be used, to diagnose or treat any medical condition. For diagnosis or treatment of any medical problem, consult your own health care professional. The publishers and author are not responsible for any specific health or allergy needs that may require medical supervision and are not liable for any damages or negative consequences from any treatment, action, application or preparation, to any person reading or following the information in this book. References are provided for informational purposes only and do not constitute endorsement of any websites or other sources.

Dedication Page

"There is a light that shines beyond all things on earth, beyond us all, beyond the heavens, beyond the very highest, the very highest heavens.
This is the light that shines in our hearts."
~ *Chandogya Upanishad*

This book is dedicated to my students who continue to teach me that the answers are found within themselves. Without you, I'd have no one to share my light with.
To my husband, who allows my light to shine in all its' "crazy wonderful colors." Your support and encouragement has been my greatest gift. You are truly my guru.
To Martin Kirk, I have only sincere adoration and heartfelt thanks for your teachings.
To my editor Gail Powell, thank you for teaching me to slow down.
To all those who continue to light up the world for others to follow: May you continue to experience many things that both humble and hearten your resolve.
Keep shining and keep opening the hearts of others!

saha nau avatu
saha nau bhunaktu
saha veeyam karavaavahi
tejasvi nau adheetam astu
ma vidvishaavahai

May we be protected *(the teacher and the student)*
May we be prosperous *(together)*
May we be strengthened *(together)*
May what we study be effective and powerful
May we not dislike each other

Introduction

"*Be a spot on the ground, where nothing is growing,*
where something might be planted, a seed, from the Absolute."
~ Tao Proverb

In a time where the meaning of yoga in the Western world has become yet another way to exercise and the push to make yoga a business has materialized, instructors today must rise up and re-connect with the hearts of their students. We must revisit our purpose for teaching yoga and redefine our interpretation of this ancient practice.

I believe any person who takes their first step on the mat has done so for the simple reason to find or create change in their lives. Whether that change is a physical one; a change in habits; thinking or relating; yoga has proven to be an important first step. As more people seek to find happiness, there's a longing in their hearts to open. As a yoga instructor, it's important to create a safe environment to facilitate this heart awakening. It could be in the music you play, the soft tone of your voice, or the meditation you provide before they slip into Savasana *(corpse pose)*. How ever they get there, welcome them to your class and teach them to sing from their heart.

As instructors we all know that in Sanskrit, Yuj translates into *yoga* and means *to yoke, or to join.* But what is it that we are really joining? We are essentially joining the light in our hearts together. We are coming together in happiness, joy and love to make the world a better place.

One of the goals in yoga is to understand that we are part of one source. We are all related. All connected. Our goal in life is to realize that it is our true inherent nature to be in service of this light and love. If the absolute *One* is light and love, and we are "all one", then we are also "light and love." How do we know this to be true? The same way The *One* knows itself to be true: it creates a cloak (a veil of darkness), then experiences everything it is *not* in order to realize what it *is*: light and love. The true meaning and path of yoga is to realize that we are not merely a *mother*, a *father*, a *CEO, a Bill or a Janet*, we are all beings of light and love, all part of the infinite *One; Brahma, The Source, God* or *Spirit* (whatever your perception of The *One* is). We forget *what* we are (light and love) and rather put *who* we are into emphasis. The goal of yoga is to open the heart of the student so that they can have an awakening to a higher revelation of *what* they truly are, rather than *who* they think they are. We are born of love, happiness and joy. This is our primary nature. It's our life experience and societal persuasions that shape us as people, yet our soul remains the same. The light from our soul ignites within and is always flickering but sometimes dim. Often the cloaks we wear are so heavy and dark that they snuff out the light in our hearts. Yoga practice is meant to *turn on the light* inside of all of us so that we can be reminded that our hearts are full of this light and love and that we are all part of that *One* infinite source: *One love and One light.*

Today it seems that some of us have forgotten that yoga is a system of revealing and remembering. Instead, we've created an exercise system for our outer bodies to achieve physical improvement. Which yes, *is* healthy because exercise in general releases chemicals in our brains such as endorphins and serotonin and yes, make us feel happier and better about ourselves in the short term, but what about the bigger picture? Why is yoga so good for our spiritual selves? Where and when is this being taught? How does the yoga instructor open the hearts of the student in order to bring about this remembering?

If you have studied *The Yoga Sutras of Patanjali*, you would have learned that yoga is an eight-step process that's studied by many on the path to enlightenment: the attainment of spiritual knowledge or insight. This process is divided into four Padas (sections). The first Pada is Samadhi Pada in which Patanjali describes this yoga path: the nature and means to attain bliss. Next is Sadhana Pada where Patanjali teaches of practice or discipline. Vibhuti Pada describes super normal powers (that can be achieved through yoga) and how to avoid misuse of these powers. Kaivalya Pada is isolation and the process of liberation and transcending the ego to become one with The Divine. The sutras barely mention the word asana *(yoga postures)*. So why do we as yoga instructors put the most emphasis on the physical asana? Perhaps we're on our own journey of awakening and remembering.

Recall the first time you stepped on a mat, what feelings and emotions did you experience during and especially after the class? Physically, you probably felt happier, sat taller and breathed more deeply. But what happened in the next hour or so after the class? Was your drive home calmer? Did you feel like you were walking on air? Did your stress levels go down? The spiritual residual felt upon leaving your first yoga class made you want to come back. So how do you extend that yoga peacefulness for more than an hour after a yoga class? By beginning to instill an opening in the heart.

The more your heart opens, the more the heart opens you. It's like the grime on the bathroom mirror. It's difficult to see who you truly are at first. After wiping it for a moment, you may get glimpses here and there of your true reflection. When you continue to wipe down the mirror, you can see a bit more clearly. The more you wipe, the clearer it gets. It takes patience but eventually it becomes unblemished for you to see your true reflection.

The concept of yoga as exercise is a good place to start, however to further deepen the practice for those ready to consider the true path to yoga, is to remember *what* we truly are: light and love.

What makes us want to share this practice with others? How do we as yoga instructors open the hearts to remembrance? By asking the question: "*What makes your heart sing?*"

How do you make the heart sing? *By threading spiritual and physical attributes into your yoga classes through theme.*

Sanskrit used in the Introduction

Savasana – corpse pose

Brahma – the Hindu god of creation

Patanjali (Tamil) – is the complier of the Yoga Sutras, a collection of aphorisms (sayings) on yoga practice

Pada – feet

Samadhi – bliss

Sadhana – practice or discipline

Vibhuti – power or manifestation

Kaivalya – isolation

Chapter One:
Make a Meaningful Connection

"Just as a flower gives out its fragrance to whomsoever approaches or uses it,
so love from within us radiates toward everybody
and manifests as spontaneous service."
~ *Swami Ramdas*

Class themes can include conscientious sharing of personal life lessons. It's about showing vulnerability as an instructor and as a person. Shine the lighter side of your personality and truly relate to your students.

A theme doesn't have to be complicated, nor long and arduous. It can be as simple as reading a quote, sharing a personal story or teaching a part of yoga philosophy. Themes are used to teach something more than the physical side of yoga.

Making tangible connections for your participants with the postures in your yoga class and the words you say will help you reach out to an individual's natural learning preference.

American author and poet Henry David Thoreau said: *"If a man does not keep pace with his companions, perhaps it's because he hears a different drummer, let him step to the music he hears, however measured and far away."*

Stepping to the music *he* hears. Everyone processes information at different frequencies. To teach only asana, is to teach only stretching and strengthening. Theming a class will make meaningful connections to the hearts, bodies and spirits of every individual in the room. Joy, happiness and love will increase because the students have been able to contemplate the lesson you provide and carry this with them throughout the day. Their calmness will be shared and peace will be created.

A theme is the connection piece: it's a link to the heart, the inner light that shines in all of us. It creates a sense of oneness with the body, the spirit and community. Students may leave your class feeling closer to enlightenment. And in turn perhaps share their knowledge with others. They will then pay it forward.

How rewarding is that?

As the instructor, you will light the spark that ignites the light for others to find their way out of the darkness. And it all begins with a theme....

Chapter Two:
Why Theme?

"At the end of the way is freedom. Till then, patience."
~ *Buddha*

When practicing yoga with an injury it's difficult to let go the thought of a posture causing pain. The natural tendency is to hold on tight while assessing the limitation when attempting the asana. But this creates tension in the body.

Years ago I had injured my lower back and was later diagnosed with two slipped discs. Sometimes I would wake in pain and spend the morning crying before putting on a brave face to teach my own yoga classes. At other times, the slipped discs would pinch my sciatic nerve and I'd have trouble even moving my leg. While I coped with the numbness and pain for two years, I would leave class feeling tense and agitated because I was so afraid that I would tweak something and cause myself more pain. My mind would not let go of the fear, and the energy I directed toward the injury seemed to feed it and give it life. As I searched outside myself for help to ease the pain, a little voice inside my head said that I already had the answers. I would use yoga to heal myself. As I began to strengthen my core and back muscles with yoga, I began to feel stronger and I knew I needed to seek a more a therapeutic approach to my practice. However, I still felt as though there was something missing.

On my healing journey, I experienced a revelation about opening my heart at a weekend yoga workshop. We'd already worked through a number of things emotionally in order to access the ability to let go through yoga practice. During our morning session the instructor taught us about Eka Rasa (one essence) and its meaning. She taught us that every emotion we experience has a deep underlying desire to feel love. With cello music softly playing in the background, our class began with a series of postures that built heat and opened our shoulders and hips. It was as though I could feel the sound of the cello deep within my heart. With the gentle guidance of her voice plucking at my heartstrings, I prepared for our peak pose. It was the pose I feared the most: Urdhva Dhanurasana (wheel pose.)

With our bodies warmed, and our minds focused, I placed my hands beside my ears, palms down, first up onto my head, then widened my arms, and set my shoulders into their sockets. I listened to the instructor's voice guide me through the process. I curled my heart up and then I let go of the physical part of the pose and worry that I had been holding in my lower back. I could feel the tips of my shoulder blades lift my heart and I straightened my arms. Up I went.

Then it happened…CRACK! Like when a baby chick bursts forth from its egg, my heart burst open and I felt elation. "Holy shift!" I said, as I came down. That felt so good in my heart. I was surprised by the lack of tightness in my lower back and no pinching. As a matter of fact, I didn't even think about my back injury, all I could hear was the instructor's voice saying, "Every emotion has a deep longing to experience love." And I really wanted to feel love – love for myself, love for my practice – that Eka Rasa she spoke of. Down again and up two more times. I couldn't stop myself. I did Urdhva Dhanurasana four times! My heart was so open, my back was safe and my physical body was strong. My body supported my release and allowed me to really feel the pose and truly connect with my intentions of feeling love. Finally! I let go of the fear of tweaking my back and suffering the rest of the weekend. I got it!

I wondered how I was able to feel so supported and so unafraid to try Urdhva Dhanurasana in this particular class, this particular weekend. There was something magical happening to me both on and off the mat. I soon realized that the *instructor's constant reassurance about Eka Rasa and that longing in our hearts to feel love helped me connect to my body in a way I had never experienced before.*

Then it hit me: The instructor's use of a solid theme, her compassionate voice and her choice of music helped me to get out of my head and back into my heart.

Without the guiding, gracious hand of theming in yoga, I would not be practicing nor teaching today. This powerful mind/body connection that I continue to feel when doing such postures like Urdhva Dhanurasana helps me to let go of physical apprehensions and boost my heart high into the air.

This was one of my personal stories and it shows the power of themes and the importance of connecting with the heart of each student.

The power of feeling love and letting go when mixed with proper alignment and a solid theme will change your practice (and your life) for good. Trust your heart. It knows the way.

Today, I use my learning process, my studies of yoga philosophies/scripture and my own personal stories as themes to connect with my students. I create a supportive, safe and open-learning environment. I show a vulnerable side when I write/speak of my journey. I consider each student and their individual needs in my class and create a sequence that links with my theme. I've learned to open my heart with my students so that I can share the wonder and beauty of this practice called yoga.

You will learn that it is important for a yoga instructor to create a safe space to facilitate this heart awakening. Creating theme in your yoga class is a very effective way to create this positive environment that will assist your participants in making tangible connections to both you and to themselves.

As you begin to open the hearts of your students, you will be creating a shift in consciousness. This is a great reflection on you, the instructor, to bring forth more joy and happiness to those in your class. Subtle themes can be interlaced into your class with ease. Students already reap the benefits of stretching and strengthening through asanas and creating greater lung capacity through guided breathing. Now, by adding the spiritual/emotional component that wipes away more grime on the mirror, you will tune into their hearts and help them see themselves more clearly.

As yoga instructors, you will learn to theme your classes using a model that includes a lesson plan designed to target four types of learning preferences. You will have a brief overview of each learning preference, their character traits and what portion of your class lesson plan relates to them. As you develop your lessons and themes, you will be able to connect with your entire class and to each and every student in the room using this simple method…and soon, hearts will sing!

Sanskrit used in Chapter Two

Urdhva Dhanurasana – wheel pose
Eka Rasa – one essence

Chapter Three:
Learning Preferences

"If you do not compare yourself with another you will be what you really are."
~ Krishnamurti

When yoga journeyed to the West, it became apparent that bigger classes would serve the masses. The yoga trend continues to turn this once fringe practice into studios filled to capacity. Your class will likely consist of more than one person so it will be helpful to be able to read the needs and learning preferences of each student. Knowing your audience and being able to read each student as they walk through the door is a learned skill that comes with experience and practice. It's necessary as a teacher to be skilled in the art of reading a diverse group of people in such a short period of time. Students will arrive with either an open heart or a closed heart. Some may come from a home with little support and then enter a yoga studio, to find a kula *(a community of the heart)* is waiting for them.

I've adapted Four Learning Preferences to help yoga instructors connect with the unique hearts of their students. These learning preferences are based on: American educational theorist, David Kolb's Learning Styles: Active Experimentation (doing), Concrete Experience (feeling), Reflective Observation (watching), and Abstract

Conceptualization (thinking); Dr. Bernice McCarthy's 4MAT learning models and The Center for Accelerated Learning's SAVI major modes of learning: Somatic (learn by physical activity), Auditory (talking and social interaction), Visual (watching and listening), and Intellectual (reflecting, thinking and analyzing).

The Four Learning Preferences (4LP's)

Each learning preference asks four inquiry questions:

1. Learning Preference One (LP1) "Why am I here?"
2. Learning Preference Two (LP2) "What am I learning, accomplishing?"
3. Learning Preference Three (LP3) "How do I apply this learning?"
4. Learning Preference Four (LP4) "What if I share this?"

LP1: "Why am I here?"
These students are the auditory learners. They are social and reflective. They're usually the ones who have been dragged to class by a friend who absolutely loves yoga. They tend to be the skeptics. They like to make an entrance and be acknowledged. They need to know *why* they should begin this journey, and how it relates to them. They may tell their story (and perhaps be a little negative at first – this is out of fear) as they seek out like-minded people in the class. They resist change when you first hit an emotional chord with them and begin to take the darkness out of their hearts. Once they feel comfortable they will then share their ideas with others in order to create a sense of harmony within the group. When their hearts finally open, they will be your best ambassadors: creating harmony, expressing genuine concern for others, and by cultivating kula.

LP2: "What am I learning, accomplishing?"
These are the intellectual students. They are sequential thinkers. They will be very aware of their bodies, perhaps athletic and involved with sports. They come to class with a specific goal such as building strength and stamina. They will want to know the benefits of each posture and what it does physically in their bodies. They are eager learners who will understand alignment and anatomy. However, they will be least interested in the spiritual connection. They may or may not like the hidden message in your theme as it will get them to realize that they are more than just a

human being, and that yoga is more than a physical exercise, so be aware of their resistance to the opening of their hearts. They need time to think things through (holding postures longer), taking facts and forming theories.

LP3: "How do I apply this learning?"
These students are the visual and tactile learners. Similar to LP2 these students will want information about postures, however only in bits and pieces. They will understand and grasp the concepts (such as alignment principles). They are hands-on people. They do not tolerate unclear ideas, as they are results driven. They like to know the plan. You can advance these students with demonstrations and physical adjustments. They will benefit from the spiritual teachings and life lessons that come from making their hearts sing. Their motto, *If it works for me, I'll use it!*

LP4: "What if I share this?"
These students are the risk takers and seek to influence others by bringing action to new ideas and concepts. They take what works to make it better. They have the courage to try new things and understand the *bigger* picture. They will add their positive feedback and share their own ideas about your lesson. They love trial and error and believe in self-discovery. They are flexible (in mind) and adaptable. You can use these people wisely in your class when demonstrating postures. They will encourage and influence others. They want to teach the world to sing from their hearts by sharing what they have learned.

Coming Full Circle

> *"When you see that everything is different, that everything is unique,*
> *you become one with the whole."*
> *~ Swami Prajnanpad*

When you learn to write and formulate a class lesson plan and create theme, you are taking into consideration four learning preferences, four personality types and four inquiry questions. You are creating an experiential learning environment rather than a linear one. Just as you may prefer to read in silence, others prefer to read with music softly playing in the background or listen to audio books while someone else might prefer to read aloud.

As with all learning styles, each student will open their hearts in different ways.

LP1 will have an opening in their heart when they feel they have made a personal connection with you and be able to relate to you based on similar life experience. Their ego may play a part in exploring asana as they seek to know why it's relevant to them – so personal connection is the key.

LP2 will want to explore the physical aspect of the class. Alignment cues will assist them to use their bodies to reach their goals. Exploring advanced asana as a testimony to their intellectual understanding of yoga and their bodies will feed their ego causing them to think that they are practicing yoga properly. Positive encouragement and adjustments will benefit them. When you use theme to make a spiritual connection, these students may resist at first, and then change will come as they ponder, *What am I feeling in my heart?*

LP3 will want to hear the alignment cues and see the demonstrations more so than listening to a theme. Their understanding is based on "seeing and doing" so repetition of asanas is the key. They may need hands-on adjusting in order to understand the posture you are teaching. It may take some creativity on your part using previous sequences and similar themes in order to facilitate an opening in their heart. Their hearts will sing when they understand the benefit of the spiritual teachings and life lessons.

LP4 will see the bigger picture in the theme as well as the asana and will want to adapt it. They will want to own it and teach it to others. They will become the ambassadors, teaching other people what they have learned with much enthusiasm. They may even race ahead of your instruction during class so you may want to use them in your demonstration of an advanced posture. They have a clear understanding of how to make their hearts sing.

A well-structured yoga class includes all four learning preferences to benefit both you as the instructor and the students equally. Honoring each individual learning preference creates a powerful opening in the heart.

How do you facilitate this opening in the heart? It starts with a concept.

Chapter Four:
The Concept

"Since it is all too clear it takes time to grasp it."
~ *Wumen*

The concept for a yoga class is an overall view of what the class theme will be about. The concept relates to the peak pose, theme and alignment. It is the umbrella, or the bigger picture. The following examples are three ways to determine the concept: talk story, personal story and moral of the story.

Talk Story

In Hawaii, a short phrase for telling a personal story/experience to another is referred to as a *talk story.* In four or five sentences, you should be able to convey the circumstances that came together in your experience that enabled you to know something at it's core level, that one thing that was the *"Uh-huh!"* moment, that one thing that made your heart sing.

Here is an example of a talk story: *"While one of my instructors was participating in my class about the Gunas (states of nature), she realized that the subtle cues of creating heaviness in her standing leg allowed her to hold Ardha Chandrasana (half moon balance) longer and with ease. She commented on how the theme related to her and said she typically struggles with this pose until now."*

The talk story is an event that happens where you suddenly realize and fully understand something for the first time. It is an epiphany. It is an *"Uh-huh!"* moment.

What is the uh-huh moment in this talk story?

Personal Story

"On my trip back from Punta Cana with my sister and her two daughters, we were extremely stressed out and tired because we missed our connecting flight and had to scramble to find a hotel in Minneapolis on March Break at midnight. The next day, we almost missed our flight again. When we finally boarded the plane, my sister and I sat together and began reviewing our photos. As the mental fatigue and shear exhaustion set in, we started to laugh and make fun of our pictures. We laughed the whole flight, cracking jokes, making light of the situation, and finding something silly to recall about our trip. Soon the stress of the previous day had dissolved and we felt better. I learned that day to laugh at life more often."

Sharing a personal story allows the instructor to make heartfelt connections with the students.

When did you use humour to diffuse a stressful situation?

Moral of the Story

When you are trying to develop the concept for your class lesson plan by using the moral of the story method, think of the concept as the bigger picture. To capture the essence of something and to come to truly understand the core of an idea, a book, a movie, a yoga philosophy, recall the moment when everything suddenly became clear.

Imagine you just watched your favorite TV show. Someone asks you what the episode was about. Right away, you answer with a quick synopsis, cutting through all the details, the plot, the characters in it, and then wrapping it up with the ending and the moral of the story.

To determine the *Moral of the Story* try this exercise:

_____ (name of a TV show/movie/book)

a lesson in _____ (the moral of the story).

The talk story, the personal story and the moral of the story are three ways to connect to the heart of the student. As an effective yoga instructor, the atmosphere you create sets the tone for the class. Drawing upon knowledge of concept completes the formula for an effective yoga class.

Concept and Theme: A delicate balance of creation

Theme and concept is like the playful dance of creation between Shiva and Shakti as told in the RigVeda *(ancient Vedic Sanskrit hymns)*.

The dance of Shiva and Shakti is lila, the play of creation. Shiva is pure consciousness; the changeless background for which Shakti can create. Shakti is the power of Shiva that does not exist without him, nor does he exist without her. They create together.

"That One lived without breath by His self-law, there was nothing else nor aught beyond it. In the beginning, Darkness was hidden by darkness; all this was an ocean of inconscience. When the universal being was concealed by fragmentation, then by the greatness of its energy, That One was born. That moved at first as desire within, which was the primal seed of mind." ~ *RigVeda verse 10, 129, 1-5*

As the One desires to know itself, it manifests as many.

Concept and theme are much like Shiva and Shakti. They co-exist with each other, they cannot exist without each other, and they create together. Without the interchangeable understanding of concept and theme, your class lesson plan would not exist. It would be like staring at one word on a piece of paper and not knowing how to make that one word manifest into many. Creation is an eternal play of two parts that make a whole: Shiva and Shakti – concept and theme.

When you create your class lesson plan, concept and theme work together to get your message across. To make hearts sing.

Here's an exercise to identify and distinguish between concept and theme:

Take for example a class in which you will be teaching about the gunas: tamas *(dense, heavy)*, rajas *(movement)* and sattva *(calmness, clarity, balance)*. Is the concept the gunas? The concept can be one of many things, it all depends on what message you are conveying in your lesson to open the hearts of your students in any particular class.

Say for instance you wish to teach about sattva and convey calmness, and balance. You choose to do a class that incorporates balance poses. As you weave sattva, calmness and balance into your class, what is it that you're really trying to convey? What's the bigger picture? The bigger picture may be that you're asking the students to let go of inhibitions, fears, or desires in order to find stillness through balance in the message of the gunas. *Hmmm, finding stillness through balance. That's quite a concept!*

So, the concept is: Finding Stillness Through Balance. The theme is the *gunas* (sattva in particular). You weave the theme of the gunas into your class through your concept. Both concept and theme are interchangeable.

You can start the class by defining the gunas. Teach students to feel heaviness, movement and stillness in their asana practice as you weave your theme (gunas) into your class through the concept (finding stillness through balance) by teaching sattva. Emphasize sattva in their bodies (or minds) by encouraging them to explore stillness in a balance asana such as Vrksasana *(tree pose)*.

Now you have three effective ways to determine your concept: a talk story, a personal story and the moral of the story.

Next, you will choose your asana, sequence and music (if any) and write The Opening and The Closing.

The following chapters will teach you how to choose asana and build a sequence while weaving your theme into your class.

Sanskrit used in Chapter Four

RigVeda – ancient Vedic Sanskrit hymns
Gunas – states of nature
Ardha Chandrasana – half moon balance pose
Shiva – pure consciousness
Shakti – power of creation
Tamas – dense, heavy, inertia
Rajas – movement
Sattva – calmness
Vrksasana – tree pose

Chapter Five:
How Do You Choose a Theme?

"Quiet the outgoing mental restlessness and turn the mind within.
…Then you will see the underlying harmony in your life and in all nature."
~ Paramahansa Yogananda

Start simple. What made your heart sing today? What made you feel happy?

If you are having challenges answering those questions then choose a yoga philosophy, a poem, a saying or a quote that resonates with you as your inspiration for your theme. Maybe share a personal story or borrow another's story. Make it simple and teach what you know. If you have not yet studied Patanjali's Yoga Sutras, then you may lack the confidence to teach about yamas *(ethical rules)* and niyamas *(restraints)*.

If you have not yet learned the lesson yourself, then the lesson is not ready to be shared. Turn on your light and find what makes your heart sing.

Here are some simple questions to ask yourself to help you choose a theme:

What made you smile today?
What made you laugh or feel happy?
Did someone do something kind for you recently?
Did you do something kind for someone else?
Have you watched an inspirational video/TV show/documentary?
What lesson have you learned lately?
Did someone post an inspirational quote on social media that spoke to you?
Do you have a favorite quote?
What in nature makes you smile, feel good, or happy?
Who or what do you love?

You can also use themes from yoga philosophy. Here are a few ideas:

Any of Patanjali's Yoga Sutras
Avidya *(incorrect knowledge)*
Kanchukas *(cloaks or veils)*
Chakras *(energy centers along the spinal column)*
Any of the Narada Bhakti Sutra *(the process of devotion)*
Duhkha *(suffering)* Sukha *(happiness)*
Gunas *(states of nature)*
Eka Rasa *(one essence)*
Bhagavad Gita *(a 700-verse Dharmic scripture)*
Shiva *(a Hindu deity – The Transformer, The Destroyer)*
The Ramayana *(ancient story portraying characters like the ideal father, ideal servant, the ideal brother, the ideal wife and the ideal king)*

Another way to choose a theme is by the process of "mind dumping" which is a fast and effective way to get a lot of information from your mind to your paper or computer. It's a great place to start when choosing a theme for your class lesson plan. By talking out loud, jotting down ideas (in no particular order), you can brainstorm and draw inspiration from your yoga practice, life experiences and knowledge.

Workbook Exercise

When you recalled the first time you stepped onto a yoga mat (in the introduction of this book) reflect on how it felt. Use the space below to practice a Mind Dumping exercise.
Write about your experience:

Your words, pictures, and feelings all tell a story. Once you have your story you can begin to develop your theme. What makes you want to share this yoga experience with others? Perhaps, you wish for others to feel as *content* as you did. So the theme for this class can be: Contentment.

In order to be effective in making hearts sing, we must remember whom it is we are teaching. As the format of the class starts to take shape within this system you will see, if followed correctly, how you will be able to open the hearts of all students.

In the beginning, you may choose to use the same theme and just change the asanas within the class to encourage an opening in the heart. When your heart sings, it creates love. So ask yourself: *What do you love?* Now relate that same feeling of love to those around you. Share the opening in your heart to make a meaningful connection to the four learning preferences. *When the lamp of light within your heart opens, it shines the light for the rest to follow.*

Chapter Six:
Basic Structure of a Yoga Class

*"Build this day on a foundation of pleasant thoughts. Never fret at any imperfec-
tions that you fear may impede your progress. Remind yourself, as often as necessary, that you are a creature of God and have the power to achieve any dream by
lifting up your thoughts. You can fly when you decide that you can. Never consider
yourself defeated again. Let the vision in your heart be in your life's blueprint."*
~ *Og Mandino*

This chapter includes templates that can be used as guidelines when creating a
sequence for a beginner class and an intermediate/advanced class. Alternatively,
you can use your preferred sequence style when creating your class lesson plan.

Basic Guidelines for Beginner classes

The Opening – what you say to make a connection to the participants in your class

Seated Centering

Warm Up – facilitating movements in the big joints, big muscles first

Heat Building Sequence – can be in the form of Surya Namaskar *(sun salutations)* or standing asana

Standing Asana – builds heat in the body

Standing Balance Asana

Twisting Asana

Seated Asana

Cool Down – forward folds

Inversions

The Closing – what you say to anchor the lesson

Relaxation – Savasana

Begin with **LP1: "Why am I here?"**
LP1 needs to be engaged first, otherwise they will lose interest, try to seek attention and may become disruptive in class. You will make a harmonious connection to the LP1 learning preference when you reveal your theme, tell your story or read a quote in The Opening.

LP2: "What am I learning, accomplishing?"

LP2 will become more engaged when the dynamic movements of the asanas begin. They will feel empowered when you cue alignment and allow them to explore their own bodies. They may not understand the theme at first, but they will understand the physical postures. Remember, they may already have knowledge of asana, so hands-on corrections to get them aligned properly will be your focus with this learning preference. Anything that's new to them will keep them interested.

LP3: "How do I apply this learning?"

LP3 will be engaged when they can see, feel and do the asana. They will be receptive to hearing the theme gently woven throughout the class as a subtle reminder. They will benefit from watching the demonstrations. Gentle hands-on adjusting is beneficial to this learning preference as they may need to feel physical alignment of their bodies.

LP4: "What if share it?"

LP4 will be immediately engaged in the asanas and the theme. They will hear and quickly understand the theme and verbal cues and will want to accelerate their practice. The Closing will anchor the lesson for the LP4 learning preference as they reflect to themselves, *What if I could take this lesson with me and show others?*

The whole concept is brought back full circle for everyone with The Closing (the quote or saying you use to anchor your theme). This process will invite all students to take what they've learned and experienced in your class off the mat and into the world. The little lights in their hearts will start to flicker!

Each movement, each word, each breath will bring about a change in the energy fields of all four learning preferences. This is why it is important to continually weave your theme subtly throughout the class. You never know when you are going to be the catalyst or the container for them when the light comes on in their hearts and they begin to sing.

Basic Guidelines for Intermediate and Advanced classes

The Opening – what you say to make a connection to the participants in your class

Seated Centering

Warm Up

Shoulder Opener

Heat Building Sequence

Core Sequence – optional

Standing Asana

Balance Asana

Peak Pose – the apex of your sequence

Twisting Asana

Seated Asana

Cool Down

Inversions

The Closing – what you say to anchor the lesson

Relaxation – Savasana

Chapter Seven:
"Easy as PIE" (Putting Into Effect)

"When understanding is born in me, compassion is also born."
~ Thich Nhat Hanh

Creating a class lesson plan is like baking a pie. I call it: Putting Into Effect (PIE). When you bake a pie, you have to follow a recipe. You need ingredients and tools then you have to assemble it.

First decide what kind of pie you want to make (theme)
Then choose which brand you want to use (concept)
Next gather the ingredients you need (asana and alignment)
Finally follow the instructions (formatting and sequencing)

The following example illustrates how the simple PIE method works. The lesson is about pratyahara *(withdrawal of the senses)*. We'll use the moral of the story method to determine the concept. Our peak pose will be Kurmasana *(tortoise)*.

What does pratyahara teach us? To withdraw from our senses – to go within – to experience moving inward mentally as you withdraw from the outside world, just as a tortoise withdraws into its' shell.

During the class, I will reiterate the feelings of drawing inward. I will encourage the students to move, feel and reflect on the sensations that they are feeling, and to soften in the pose as they continue to withdraw from their senses like a tortoise.

The moral of the story: Withdrawal of the Senses: a lesson in pratyahara

When formatting your lesson plan for a class, you may first write The Opening and The Closing (Step One and Step Four) then write the sequence (Step Two and Step Three). Or write the sequence first, then practice it, then discern from your sequence what it is you want to convey to open the heart of the student and then write The Opening and The Closing.

In the pratyahara lesson, I wrote The Opening and The Closing first. I knew my peak pose was tortoise, and I already knew the theme: Withdrawal of the Senses.

It was written like this:

The Opening: *"Tortoise withdraws into its shell when it is startled or threatened. When you take the form of a tortoise, you will often experience a feeling of moving inward mentally. Pratyahara means sense withdrawal. As your senses withdraw from outside distractions, your mind is less agitated and you feel centered. In our class today, we will cultivate the inner withdrawal by taking the form of Kurmasana (tortoise pose)."*

The Closing: *"When you develop the ability to stay neutral in the face of a difficult situation, you can better assess your choices and you will respond with clearer knowledge and an open heart rather than emotional conflict and reactivity."*

Next I wrote the sequence. (Step Two and Three)

Sequence:
Marjarisana-Bitilasana – cat/cow warm up
Surya Namaskar A – to build up heat
Utkatasana – to teach how to open the hips and widen the sit bones
Garudasana
Uttanasana – widen the sit bones
Adho Mukha Svanasana
Parsvakonasana – open the hips
Parighasana
Marichyasana – hug the midline
Baddha Konasana – open the hips
Upavistha Konasana – open the hips
Kurmasana – withdraw the senses
Dandasana
Setu Bandha Sarvangasana
Sukha Balasana
Savasana

When the sequence is built first and your alignment focus is in place, practice the class and then write The Opening and The Closing. In Chapter Eight, you will use a PIE format to practice writing a class lesson plan.

Sanskrit used in Chapter Seven

Pratyahara – to withdraw the senses

Kurmasana – tortoise pose

Marjarisana-Bitilasana – cat/cow warm up

Utkatasana – powerful pose (also called chair pose)

Garudasana – eagle pose

Uttanasana – forward fold pose

Parsvakonasana – extended side angle pose

Parighasana – gate-keeper pose

Marichyasana I – sage Marichi's pose

Baddha Konasana – bound angle pose

Upavistha Konasana – seated angle pose

Dandasana – staff pose

Setu Bandha Sarvangasana – bridge pose

Sukha Balasana – happy baby pose

Chapter Eight:
The PIE Format

"Practice becomes firmly established when it has been cultivated uninterruptedly
and with devotion over a prolonged period of time."
~ *Patanjali's Yoga Sutra, 1.14*

Imagine you're planning a dinner party for you and four friends. For dessert you decide to bake a pie taking into consideration each of your friends' taste preferences, favourite foods and food allergies (4LP's). You search online for a recipe (research your theme), gather the ingredients (create the concept), and now you're ready to bake the pie (write your class lesson plan).

The following workbook exercise is designed to take you through the steps for creating a class lesson plan.

Remember the first time you made cookies or baked a pie? You carefully followed a recipe step-by-step. Through trial and error, you became familiar with the method, and over time adapted the recipe to suit your preference.

Workbook Exercise

From the Mind Dumping exercise in Chapter Five, use the theme you created to make your own brand of PIE by following this exercise:

Key Components

What type of PIE? (**Theme:** What are you trying to convey? What life lesson or philosophy do you want to share?)

What brand? (**Concept:** What's the *bigger picture* of the theme? How did this story/philosophy make your heart sing? What was your *"Uh-huh!"* moment?)

What do we need? (Key ingredients in the form of asana and alignment principles. Use a separate sheet of paper to Mind Dump the asanas you will include in your sequence.

What instructions do we follow? (Formatting and sequencing. Is this a beginner, intermediate or advanced class? Follow the information provided in the **Guidelines for Basic Structure of a Class** in Chapter Six.)

Now that you have gathered the key components for your PIE, you'll begin to measure out the ingredients. Use the following space to write out your class lesson plan.

Next you will assemble the whole PIE using the template provided. If you require more space to write, you can use a separate sheet of paper.

Step One: Write The Opening

Step Two: Write your asana sequence, **Step Three:** Write your alignment principles and verbal cues. (These steps are interchangeable and often written together.)

Step Four: Write The Closing

As formatting a class lesson plan begins to take shape you will have to tools to theme an effective heart opening for all of your students. The next question is: *When and where do you weave theme?*

Chapter Nine:
Weaving Theme

*"When you move amidst the world of sense, free from attachment and aversion
alike, there comes the peace in which all sorrows end,
and you live in the wisdom of the Self."*
~ *The Bhagavad Gita*

Weaving theme is not as hard as it seems. (Remember you can always re-state your theme in The Opening and The Closing of your class).

Let's look at Withdrawal of the Senses: a lesson in pratyahara once again so that we can learn where in our sequence to weave theme.

As stated earlier pratyahara teaches us to withdraw from our senses – to go within – to experience moving inward mentally as you withdraw from the outside world, just as a tortoise withdraws into its shell.

I also stated that during the class, I reiterate the feeling of withdrawing from the senses. I will encourage the students to move, feel and reflect on the sensations that they are feeling, and to soften their bodies as they continue to withdraw from their senses like a tortoise.

Let's look at all of this information and highlight the attributes that I want to communicate during the class:
feeling resistance…moving inward mentally…softening…feeling and reflecting on sensations…withdrawing from the senses.

Let's take the following sequence and decide where to weave in the theme.

Start with feeling resistance. Where would you teach that? Then continue picking the attributes you want to teach, using all or just a few from the list. Remember, that if it's a beginner class and the students have never done yoga before, too much talking/theme/alignment may be overwhelming.

Marjarisana-Bitilasana – cat/cow warm up (maybe start in table or child's pose and teach hardness, like a tortoise's shell)
Surya Namaskar A – to build heat
Utkatasana – teach to feel resistance in the legs
Garudasana – teach alignment
Uttanasana – teach alignment and the feeling of being stuck (hamstrings are tight)
Adho Mukha Svanasana – get them to move, feel and reflect on sensations
Parsvakonasana – remain reflective - teach alignment
Parighasana – remain neutral - teach alignment (hugging in to prep for twist)
Marichyasana I – teach to withdraw from the senses and not be fearful of twisting
Baddha Konasana – teach alignment and soften groins
Upavistha Konasana – teach alignment and soften again
Kurmasana – teach alignment and to withdraw by remaining non reactive to sensations. Move inward mentally as your outer world becomes "out of focus." What you need is not out there, just like the tortoise knows that when he goes into his shell, he doesn't need the help of anyone to protect him. His protection comes from within.
Dandasana
Setu Bandha Sarvangasana
Sukha Balasana

Savasana

Usually after the peak pose Kurmasana (tortoise) as in this case, you can just teach alignment and form and then reiterate your theme in The Closing. If it feels natural to add part of your theme after the peak pose, then by all means, do so.

Now that you have the basic foundation around theming established, Chapter Ten will further explain how to put it all into effect (assemble a PIE).

Chapter Ten:
Assemble a PIE

The Gunas PIE

Let's refer to the gunas lesson from Chapter Four. When I wrote this class lesson plan, I chose poses to teach heaviness (tamas), movement and breath (rajas), hugging the midline (the general principle for balancing asanas), and standing balance asana (to teach sattva). I wrote The Opening and The Closing first based on the gunas theme, then I wrote the asana sequence. I then interlaced tamas, rajas and sattva throughout the body of the asana sequence. The alignment cues were added during the process to emphasize the theme.

Step One:

The Opening: Tell your story about the gunas here (explaining the philosophy or just define rajas, tamas and sattva).

Seated Centering

Warm Up: Get the students to feel the movement of mind and breath. Feel heavy through the foundation. Now find the balance between movement, heaviness and stillness.

Step Two (asana) and Step Three (alignment):

The Sequence: (interweaving theme, alignment principles and asana).
Use tamas to create the heaviness needed as you root your feet firmly into the earth. Allow rajas, movement to occur for a moment, then teach them to find the balance between heavy and movement, thus creating stillness and balance: sattva.

Remember to follow the basic structure of a yoga class. You can do it this way:

Teach Tadasana – weave tamas and rajas in Tadasana.

Lift one leg – teach standing balance alignment and weave tamas, rajas then sattva to find balance through stillness.

Lunge – can teach tamas, rajas then do floating lunge to teach sattva.

Vinyasa through Plank, Chaturanga Dandasana, Bhujangasana, Adho Mukha Svanasana, Uttanasana up to Tadasana.

Lunge – teach as per above but then transition into T-Pose balance (to show the form of Virabhadrasana III).

Vinyasa to Tadasana as per above.

Virabhadrasana I – teach the form (alignment), teach tamas, rajas, then do Virabhadrasana III, weaving tamas, rajas then sattva to find the balance in stillness. Vinyasa to Tadasana as per above.

You can teach Virabhadrasana II and turn it into Ardha Chandrasana – this can be your peak pose (I personally structured a class like this and one of my instructors was attending. She commented that she has never felt so free, stable or strong in her Ardha Chandrasana as she did that day. What an accomplishment on both our parts – what did she learn differently that allowed her to experience this? Could it have been alignment cues? Or perhaps it was the whole finding balance where she felt she had none?)

Finish with a seated twist, forward fold, supine asana, gentle inversion and then Savasana.

Step Four:

The Closing: In Savasana you can teach them to find movement in the breath as they inhale, feel heavy as they sink into the earth on the exhale, repeat a few times. Then introduce sattva, allowing them to remain in the calmness and stillness, thus finding balance through the stillness of the breath. Reiterate how through the craziness of movement of mind (think of how crazy it is when the wind is blowing things around), there is a sense of calmness in our lives when we can firmly plant our feet into the earth and find the heaviness and stability. Sometimes we just need to be still in order to find balance (perhaps share a quote that relates to this theme of finding balance through stillness).

Just like baking a PIE, you can see that creating theme is simple when you follow the recipe. However, if you forget to weave your theme throughout your class because you are focused on teaching alignment, don't worry, it takes practice. Just make sure you have a strong opening and strong closing that opens their hearts to the bigger picture.

What if you had a peak pose in mind that you wanted to create a theme for? In Chapter Eleven we will explore how to format a lesson around a peak pose.

Sanskrit used in Chapter Ten

Tadasana – mountain pose

Chaturanga Dandasana – 4 limbed staff pose

Bhujangasana – cobra pose

Adho Mukha Svanasana – downward facing dog pose

Virabhadrasana III – warrior three pose

Vinyasa – to flow

Virabhadrasana I – warrior one pose

Chapter Eleven:
Peak Pose Format

"The sages see life as a wheel, with each individual going round and round through birth and death. Individuals remain on this wheel so long as they believe themselves to be separate but once they realize their unity with God, then they break free."
~ *The Upanishads*

Inspiration comes in many different forms. Sometimes you see or learn a new pose, such as Eka Pada Koundinyasana I *(twisted one legged arm balance),* and you want to use it as your peak pose. To write your class lesson plan using a peak pose you will begin by building your sequence first.

A peak pose is like the climax of a story or the crest of a wave. It is also called the apex. The peak pose is a more challenging asana and is most often taught in intermediate and advanced yoga classes. Beginner yoga sequences teach more basic postures and peak pose is not necessarily used. A series of asanas are used to build up to the peak pose.

To build your sequence you have to break down the peak pose. If Eka Pada Koundinyasana I is your peak pose, then you must find poses that warm up, open and stretch the same way as the peak pose. Then build your sequence using the **Basic Structure of a Yoga Class** from Chapter Six.

In this next exercise, analyze the peak pose to create a sequence and class lesson plan with a theme.

Peak Pose: Eka Pada Koundinyasana I
Q: What type of asana is it?
A: *It's a hand balance.*

Q: What alignment cues are needed to teach a hand balance?
A: *Hug the midline, soften the heart and create core strength.*

Q: What are you doing in the final form of the pose in relation to the physical body?
A: *You are balancing on our hands, engaging your core and you are in a twist with the legs extended.*

Q: What do you have to warm up first?
A: *Big muscles and joints.*

Q: What do you have to stretch or open?
A: *Shoulders and hips need to be open, heart needs to be softened and core engaged.*

Q: What pose or poses do you see within the final pose?
A: *Chaturanga Dandasana; a twist with knees together; a twist with the legs apart.*

Q: What asana will you use to cool down? (If your peak pose is a twist then you don't choose a twist in the cool down.)
A: *You need to choose a counter pose such as a forward fold.*

Q: What level of student is this class designed for?
A: *Intermediate and advanced.*

After you have analyzed your peak pose, begin formatting your lesson. Write out your asana (Step Two) and your alignment principles, cues and theme (Step Three). Step Two and Step Three can be interchangeable.

In the following example, alignment principles are listed without the verbal cues. Verbal cues for each asana may differ according to the various styles of yoga learned today. Insert your preferred verbal cues after each asana listed in the sequence.

Warm Up: In the warm up, teach about melting the heart, which takes the head of the arm bone back, and places the shoulder blades flat on the back. Do Table and variations (opposite arm and leg extended) to teach melting the heart and to create core strength and then teach Kumbhakasana *(plank pose),* Adho Mukha Svanasana, Uttanasana. End in Tadasana at the top of the mat.

Heat Building: Teach a slow Surya Namaskar A using first 8-Point Pose to teach how to open the shoulders. Then build the sequence into Surya Namaskar A and hold Chaturanga Dandasana. Focus a bit on Chaturanga Dandasana as it is part of the form of our peak pose. Make sure your students understand how to open the shoulders by drawing the head of the arm bones back to set the shoulder into the shoulder socket; how to stretch their sternum forward; hug the arm bones in; soften the heart; and cultivate core strength. (When I learned this pose, I had my *"Uh-huh!"* moment when I realized how close my face had to be to the floor, thus resembling Chaturanga Dandasana and that is why I spend time teaching Chaturanga Dandasana at the beginning.)

Standing Asana: Lunge – to teach core strength and initiate muscular engagement in the legs that is needed for the final pose

Utthita Parsvakonasana – to open the hip

Utthita Trikonasana – to open the hip

Parsvottanasana – to teach form of Trikonasana with twist

Parivrtta Trikonasana – to teach leg form in Eka Pada Koundinyasana

Prasarita Padottanasana – to teach hugging into the midline and use feet to initiate muscular engagement

Brigid's Cross – to teach form of the legs, and a twist

Bakasana – to teach balancing on hands

Parivrtta Utkatasana – to teach the twist

Balance and Twist:
Parsva Bakasana – teach this form of the twisting hand-balance

Eka Pada Koundinyasana I – teach this peak pose (because the peak pose has a twist, end with a few more forward folds to cool the body, calm the nervous system and bring the body back to homeostasis)

Cool Down: Forward folds

Upavistha Konasana

Paschimottansana

Janu Sirsasana – gentle twist version

Janu Sirsasana – through the legs version

Inversion:

Setu Bandha Sarvangasana

Sarvangasana – calms nervous system

Apanasana

Savasana

Now that you have the asana sequence built, you need a theme.
How do you build a theme around an asana sequence? *You do a Mind Dumping.*

Mind Dumping Exercise

> *"Words can travel thousands of miles.*
> *May my words create mutual understanding and love.*
> *May they be as beautiful as gems, as lovely as flowers."*
> ~ *Thich Nhat Hanh*

Look at your peak pose. Is there a yoga philosophy or story related to it? Most yoga asanas are named after animals, deities or sages.

Practice the sequence and discern how you feel. What was challenging? What/How did you feel?

Start Mind Dumping all of your ideas about the peak pose (in no particular order): *philosophy…story…feeling liberated…feeling wrung out…unexpected fear (of falling on my face)…learned balance (fulcrum point)…was not what it seemed… gained strength…*

Build your story from the Mind Dumping exercise.

Write **The Opening:** *"I used to have a major fear of falling. When I was seven years old my aunt took me to a suspension bridge that went across a huge, deep ravine. Other people seem to cross the bridge just fine, but I freaked out halfway. People were passing by me and the bridge was swaying back and forth. I froze. I gripped the rope tightly and peered over the edge. I thought, 'I'm going to fall…I'm going to fall…there's too many people on this thing…it's going to break!' I couldn't under- stand how this suspension bridge could support the weight of all these people! I was so afraid of falling.*

As I attempt an arm balance in yoga, I sometimes feel a similar fear. I'm afraid my arms won't support me and I'll fall on my face. It wasn't until I learned how to break down a pose into steps and understand how close my face should be to the ground (as in Chaturanga Dandasana) that I was able to find my balance and perfect Eka Pada Koundinyasana I. Of course now I realize that the structure of the bridge was built to support the flow and weight of people on it and I use that understanding to help me let go of my fears."

Now that we have established and written The Opening we can determine the concept and theme: "all is not what it seems" (notice that this was in my Mind Dump exercise).

The theme for this lesson is to convey that 'when you learn to trust yourself and have the knowledge and understanding of the final outcome, you can release the fear' (this statement can be used in The Closing).

Practice the asana to determine if the theme relates to the lesson. Also, when you practice the sequence, be sure you can finish in the time allotted. You may have to reduce the Surya Namaskar A portion as you have three hand balances. Hand balances build a lot of heat on their own; so you can easily take out Surya Namaskar A but keep the Chaturanga Dandasana lesson.

Now write **The Closing:** *"All is not what it seems. When you allow fear to enter into your mind and take root in your thoughts you cannot see the forest for the trees. You are so afraid to fall until someone teaches you that the structure will not break and that it is made to hold the weight of many people. Trust in yourself that you know and understand that trying something new is scary at first, but with practice you'll be able to release the fear. Like you did today."*

Or something like that...

Let's do one more exercise to see what an entire class would look like using the PIE format. This exercise will help you successfully write your class lesson plan. I've included a template on how to structure your class lesson plan.

Sanskrit used in Chapter Eleven

Eka Pada Koundinyasana I – one leg sage Koundinya's pose variation one pose

Kumbhakasana – plank pose

Trikonasana – triangle pose

Parsvottanasana – side stretched out pose

Parivrtta Trikonasana – revolved triangle pose

Prasarita Padottanasana – wide legged forward fold pose

Bakasana – crane pose

Parivrtta Utkatasana – revolved powerful pose (chair pose with a twist)

Parsva Bakasana – revolved crow pose

Paschimottansana – seated forward fold

Janu Sirsasana – head of the knee pose

Sarvangasana – shoulder stand pose

Apanasana (Supta Balasana) – knees to chest pose (reclined baby pose)

Chapter Twelve:
Let's Make a PIE

"Offer unto me that which is very dear to thee — which thou holdest most covetable. Infinite are the results of such an offering."

~ Bhagavad Gita

Follow the steps below to write your class lesson plan. If you need more space to write, use a separate sheet of paper.

1. Read the entire sequence.
2. Answer questions A and B at the end of the sequence.
3. Condense the story or philosophy to five-to-seven sentences to write The Opening.
4. Write The Closing.
5. Determine the concept and create the theme.
6. Weave the theme into the class by choosing where in the sequence you will talk about the theme. Use the space provided to write your alignment principles and verbal cues.

When you are done this exercise, you will have a class to teach!

The Opening:

Seated Centering:

Warm Up: Uttanasana – start to teach to alignment

Anjaneyasana Prep – teach alignment, open hips

Bhekasana Prep – supine on belly – to stretch the quads

Anjaneyasana – Teach alignment, open hips

Eka Pada Dhanurasana (from all fours, opposite leg and arm) – alignment

Heat Building Sequence: Do 4 rounds of gentle Surya Namaskar A with emphasis on opening the shoulders in Bhujangasana

Bhekasana Prep - supine on belly - to stretch the quads

Alanasana - teach alignment, open hips

Eka Pada Dhanurasana - teach alignment

Standing Asana: Virabhadrasana II

Bhujangasana - more focus on alignment

Anjaneyasana - teach alignment

Eka Pada Rajakapotasana 2 prep - thigh stretch

Balance Asana: Eka Pada Bhekasana (standing) - teach alignment

Natarajasana

Uttanasana/Down Dog to transition into floor

Seated Twists: Parsva Upavistha Konasana

Cool Down: Upavistha Konasana

Janu Sirsasana

Paschimottanasana

Inversions: Setu Bandha Sarvangasana

The Closing:

Relaxation: Savasana

A. What is the peak pose?

B. Explain the philosophy or story attached to the peak pose?

Your grasp of concept and theme is beginning to take shape in your class lesson plan. Let's do a few more workbook exercises in order to open the hearts of the students using the PIE format.

Sanskrit used in Chapter Twelve

Anjaneyasana – monkey lunge pose

Bhekasana – frog pose

Alanasana – crescent lunge pose

Eka Pada Dhanurasana – one-legged bow pose

Eka Pada Rajakapotasana – one-legged pigeon pose

Eka Pada Bhekasana – one-legged frog pose

Natarajasana – dancer pose

Parsva Upavistha Konasana – lateral seated angle pose

Chapter Thirteen:
Tweaking the Ingredients

"If your compassion does not include yourself, it is incomplete."
~ Buddha

Workbook Exercise

The following exercise is designed to help you format your own PIE. Read the Hanuman (monkey god) story. Answer the questions to complete the exercise. Chapter Fourteen includes a template to help you structure your class lesson plan. If you need more space to write, you can use a separate sheet of paper.

The Story of Hanuman

Hanuman is a monkey god who is devoted to the deity: Ram. Hanuman sees the godliness in Ram even though Ram is banished from his kingdom. Ram is sent to live in the forest for 14 years. He takes his wife Sita, and his brother Lakshmana to live with him. While in the forest, Sita is kidnapped by a demon and is taken across the ocean to Lanka. Hanuman is so devoted to Ram that he vows to find Sita and bring her back. After one attempt to rescue Sita, where Hanuman grows 10 times his size to leap across the ocean, Hanuman has to return to tell Ram that Ram is the only one who can save Sita. Together, they form an army, build a bridge and cross the ocean. A battle ensues and Lakshmana is injured. Hanuman goes to the Himalayas to find herbs to heal Lakshmana. When Hanuman does not know which herb to bring back, he brings the whole mountain back. Ram and his army, along with the devoted Hanuman defeat the evil demon and rescue Sita.

Hanuman's story is a parable to life. When you recognize Divine nature of life, offer yourself to it and let it transform you in ways you never thought possible in order to serve your highest purpose. Approach your asana practice today with such conviction as Hanuman did in the story and your journey will always have a purpose.

Complete the exercise by answering the following questions:

Q: What do you think the peak pose should be?
A: Hanumanasana *(splits pose)*. This pose represents the leap across the ocean.

Q: What kind of pose is it?
A:

Q: What do you need to warm up and open?
A:

Q: What alignment do you need to teach?
A:

Q: What poses prepare the body for the final asana?

A:

Q: Where will you weave your theme?

A:

After completing this workbook exercise, use the **Build Your Sequence Template** in Chapter Fourteen to write out your class lesson plan.

Chapter Fourteen:
Build Your Sequence Template

Quick Reference Template:

The Opening

Seated Centering

Warm Up

Heat Building Sequence

Standing Asana

Balance Asana

Seated Twisting Asana

Seated Asana

Cool Down

Inversions (Setu Bandha Sarvangasana for beginners)

The Closing

Relaxation: Savasana

The Opening:

Seated Centering:

Warm Up: facilitate movements in the big joints, big muscles first (3-4 asanas)

Heat building sequence: can be in the form of Surya Namaskar (4 rounds) or standing asana (4 asanas)

Standing Asana: teach the form, weave the theme (4-5 asanas)

Balance Asana: standing (1-2 asanas)

Seated Twisting Asana: (1 asana)

Seated Asana: (1-2 asanas)

Cool Down: forward folds (2-3 asanas)

Inversions: (Setu Bandha Sarvangasana, for beginners)

The Closing:

Relaxation: Savasana

Chapter Fifteen:
Workbook Exercise Section

Workbook Exercise #1

Take the following class lesson plan and highlight with different colors the Basic Structure of a Yoga Class. For example: The Opening, Warm Up, Heat Building Sequence, Standing Asana, Standing Balance Asana, etc.

All Of My Heart

"My dog Moka is the cutest Yorkie-Poo you'll ever meet. He has such an amazing personality. When he sits on my lap and looks up at me with his puppy dog eyes, I can feel him telling me how much he loves me too. I love him so much, that I can just 'eat him up' (as I often tell him). So how does this feeling translate into every day life? There is a word in Sanskrit that means 'with all of the heart'. It is called sarvabhava. 'Sarva' means 'all' and 'bhava' means 'existing' or 'soul heart'. Sarvabhava can then translate as all of one's being or the whole of one's existence. * 'Think of what you mean when you tell a person you love that you do so 'with all of your heart'. Your love is unbounded, undiminished, true, unconditional, strong, deep, unfeigned. When you love another with all your heart, you love from the entirety of your being, from the depths of your soul.'

The way I know that Moka loves me and I love him. In your practice today, fill the heart with energy and let it pour out. Put your heart into your practice and learn to feel with the essence that is sarvabhava: all of the heart."

Table – teach alignment of hands, arms and shoulders

Anahatasana – teach to align and open shoulders and weave the theme: *"Allow your heart to melt."*

Table

Urdhva Mukha Svanasana – teach alignment of shoulders and weave the theme: *"Pour your heart into your downward facing dog."*

Uttanasana

Tadasana

Tadasana – teach with hands interlaced behind the back. Teach to lengthen the sides of the body, draw the head of the arm bones back and open the shoulders.

Uttanasana – teach with the same arm position as Tadasana. Cue lengthening the sides of the body, arm bones back and shoulder openers while weaving theme: *"Fill the heart with energy and let it pour out."*

Surya Namaskar A – teach 4 rounds and focus on shoulder openers and soften the heart in cobra.

1st Round of Surya Namaskar A – vinyasa onto the belly and teach Makarasana to teach shoulder openers, and solidify the softening of the heart at the bottom tips of the shoulder blades.

2nd Round of Surya Namaskar A – vinyasa onto belly and teach baby Bhujangasana. Use the same cues and alignment as in 1st round and weave the theme: *"Feel with all your heart."*

3rd Round of Surya Namaskar A – vinyasa onto belly and teach full Bhujangasana. Same alignment, and add more inner and outer rotation of upper femur bones to protect the lower back.

4th Round of Surya Namaskar A – vinyasa onto belly and teach Urdhva Mukha Svanasana. Teach to anchor the feet, keep the back body full (especially in the kidneys) inner and outer rotation of the femur bones as well as shoulder openers.

Vinyasa to Tadasana

Virabhadrasana I – teach shoulder openers.

Parsvakonasana – teach shoulder openers. Invite students to begin to express putting their heart into their practice.

Trikonasana – Same cues at as Parsvakonasana, with emphasis on allowing freedom to take the heart more open in a little back bend.

Prasarita Padottansana – teach lengthening the spine, head of the arm bones back, further softening the heart as you weave the theme: *"Sometimes the heart must soften in order to experience sarvabhava."*

Ardha Chandrasana – teach the form of the pose then add shoulder opener to open the heart and weave the theme: *"Fill up with as much energy as you can and let your heart shine with all of your being."*

Padattonasana – use this pose to stretch the back body after back bends.

Tadasana

Uttanasana

Urdhva Muka Svanasana – restate the theme: *"Feel with all your heart."*

Dhanurasana – teach 3 rounds.

1st Round of Dhanurasana – teach to just hold the feet, activate energy through muscle contraction, keep body aligned, and initiate shoulder openers and weave the theme: *"The more we experience love, the more we feel love."*

2nd Round of Dhanurasana – teach same alignment as 1st round, then cue them to press their feet back into their hands to feel thighs lift, notice it begins to lift the chest.

3rd Round of Dhanurasana – full pose: push feet back into the hands and cue shoulder opener to open the heart and weave the theme: *"Sarvabhava, with all my heart!"*

Pashimottanasana

Janu Sirsasana

Windshield Wipers

Apanasana

Savasana
"When we think of sarvabhava, we can picture that which we love with all of our heart; with every essence of our being. Take a few moments now to reflect on who or what it is that you love with all your heart. I ask you this: Did you include your self amongst those you love?"

*(source: *Exquisite Love: Heart-centered Reflections on the Narada Bhakti Sutras* by: William K. Mahony.)

Workbook Exercise #2

In this next class lesson example I used asana to match the yama and niyama I was teaching. I have left out the transitions in the example as you may choose to flow into the next asana or just step back from Tadasana each time.

Highlight the asanas in this class.
Living in Peace: A Lesson in Yamas and Niyamas

The Opening: *"In Patanjali's Yoga Sutras, we learn about the 8 limbs of yoga that are a part of a system used to reach enlightenment. The first two limbs teach us about our outer observances and inner restraints. They are called the yamas and niyamas. Think of these limbs as the foundational aspect to attaining bliss on our journey to wellness. Yamas and niyamas teach us about our attitudes and how we deal with people and situations and how we use our energy. Each step is meant to wipe away the grime that shrouds our hearts from experiencing love. As we practice today, we will reflect on the five yamas and five niyamas and learn how to live in peace."*

Adho Mukha Svanasana – teach ahimsa (*non-harming,* the first yama). A lot of people collapse the armpits in downward facing dog, so use this pose to create proper alignment in the shoulders. Get them to feel correct alignment to experience ahimsa.

Lunge Sequence – lunge then lunge with a twist, to Parivrtta Parsvakonasana – teach satya *(truthfulness).* With each transition, allow participants to advance their practice and to be truthful about how they feel in the pose. Is the truth they seek a need to use blocks to bring the floor closer to them?

Utkatasana – teach asteya *(non-coveting).* Be happy with your own practice thus far.

Parsva Utkatasana – teach form of the peak pose Parsva Bakasana.

Kumbhakasana – to teach form of hand balance.

Bakasana – teach brahmacharya *(sense control)*. Have participants sense the form of the pose from the rounded back, to the stretched heart to the Chaturanga Dandasana arms. Control the sense of sight and focus on the top of the mat and not your hands.

Parsva Bakasana (peak pose) – teach aparigraha *(non-stealing)*. Stealing doesn't have to be a physical action. Take quiet celebration in your own efforts and remember to let others shine as well.
Reaffirm the first 4 limbs in this peak pose: ahimsa, satya, asteya, brahmachariya.

Balasana – teach saucha *(purity: the first niyama)*. Teach about having pure and clean thoughts.

Dandasana to Purvottanasana – teach santosa *(contentment)*. Teach the students to be content with where they are in their practice and if their arms are tired encourage them to stay in Dandasana.
Eka Pada Rajakapotasana – teach tapas *(disciplined use of energy, perseverance)*. Eka Pada Rajakapotasana is an active pose and often people will rest and disengage muscular energy. Teach tapas (which also means heat) and that pigeon pose is an active pose. Keep the fire going by encouraging the activeness of muscular engagement in the legs.

Pashimottanasana – teach svadhyaya *(self-study)*. This pose is a forward fold, a great time to teach reflection: go within and reflect/study your practice.

Setu Bandha Sarvangasana – teach isvara pranidhana *(celebration of the spiritual)*. As students open their hearts in bridge pose, allow them to celebrate the light in their own hearts as an opening. A true celebration of the spirit!

Savasana

The Closing: *"Patanjali gives us the guidelines on how to deal with people (yamas) and how to use our own energy (niyamas), yet he does not really tell us how this is done. He invites us to ponder each step on our own journey of opening our hearts in our own way, on our own time. He essentially teaches us how to open our hearts to love and it begins with the self."*

Workbook Exercise #3

This detox yoga class lesson is called, "Cleaning House." You will vinyasa into each pose after you do the first five rounds of Surya Namaskar A.

Here is the asana practice. Weave the detox theme into the sequence.

Cleaning House

The Opening: *"According to Buddha, our bodies are our temples. Just as you would keep your house clean for those who reside there, you should keep your mind, body or 'soul house' clean too. There are times when we let the dusting of the shelves go an extra week, and the dishes pile up from time to time. And sometimes we eat things that we know are not feeding our bodies wisely. You scrub your house with household cleaner, but what do you do for your body? You clean your body temple or soul house with a rigorous yoga asana practice designed to build heat, stimulate fire and wring out the toxins! In our asana practice, we will be eliminating anything toxic from the mind, body and soul."*

Virasana

Bharadvajasana I

Adho Mukha Svanasana

5x Surya Namaskar A

Utkatasana into Simhasana while in Utkatasana with hands on thighs

Parivrtta Utkatasana

Anjaneyasana

Lunge with a twist

Trikonasana

Parivrtta Trikonasana

Prasarita Padottanasana

Parivrtta Prasarita Padottanasana

Virabhadrasana I

Parsvakonasana into

Ardha Chandrasana

Parivrtta Trikonasana into

Parivrtta Ardha Chandrasana

Vinyasa to Kumbhakasana – hold and do Kapalabhati Breath 3x

Knee to chest in plank – stimulate organs

Brigid's Cross

Marichayasana 3

Parivrtta Janu Sirsasana

Janu Sirsasana

Jathara Parivartanasana

Setu Bandha Sarvangasana x3

Supta Balasana

Savasana

Write **The Closing:**

Sanskrit used in Chapter Fifteen

Sarvabhava – all of my heart

Anahatasana – melting heart pose

Urdhva Mukha Svanasana – upward facing dog pose

Makarasana – crocodile pose

Ahimsa – non-violence, non-harming

Satya – truthfulness

Asteya – non-coveting

Brahmacharya – sense control

Aparigraha – non-possessiveness

Saucha – purity (the first niyama)

Santosa – contentment

Tapas – austerity, mental control

Svadhyaya – study of scripture

Isvara pranidhana – celebration of the spiritual

Virasana – hero pose

Bharadvajasana I – simple sitting twist pose

Simhasana – lion pose

Parivrtta Trikonasana – revolved triangle pose

Parivrtta Prasarita Padottanasana – revolved wide legged forward fold pose

Parivrtta Ardha Chandrasana – revolved triangle pose

Kapalabhati Breath – skull shining breath

Marichayasana 3 – sage Marichi's pose (a seated twist)

Parivrtta Janu Sirsasana – revolved head of the knee pose

Jathara Parivartanasana – reclined spinal twist (abdominal pose)

Chapter Sixteen:
What Makes My Heart Sing

This chapter contains some of my favorite class themes for reference.

Take a Stand
*(borrowed with permission from *The Age of Empowerment* by Susan Mann).

Teach a series of balancing asana with this sequence.

The Opening: * *"More people are stepping into their personal power. More people are seeing themselves for who they truly are, rather than how others have conditioned or viewed them. Our lights are shining brighter: our ego is dwindling. Greed, power, dominance and control as part of the 'old' structures are releasing. As these 'ego-driven' energies no longer exist in our energy fields they will eventually leave our society structures. Imagine a world without these attributes. Take a stand and feel with the heart, rather than think with the head!"*

Tadasana – teach the foundation and form as you weave theme: *"Take a stand right here, right now. Stand tall and rigid like the mountain."*

Tadasana – teach alignment as you weave theme: *"Begin to feel the power of one becoming two as you engage every muscle in your body. Hug closely to the midline to maintain this strength."*

Parvatanasana – hands interlaced above head to warm up shoulders.

Surya Namaskar A – 4 rounds to build heat.

Anjaneyasana – teach alignment as you weave theme: *"Feel the power of your legs, take a stand and free up the energy in the body to create the freedom your heart desires."*

Virabhadrasana I – teach the form then step into Virabhadrasana III. Teach alignment as you weave theme: *"In the face of danger, perhaps danger of falling, embrace the power of all your muscles working together to assist you in taking a stand to perform this standing balance pose."*

Virabhadrasana II into Utthita Parsvakonasana – weave theme: *"Stand like the warrior you are!"*

Trikonasana into Ardha Chandrasana – teach form and alignment and allow for freedom to express what it is they stand for.

Tadasana
Garudasana – teach the form and weave theme: *"The eagle sees with such clarity. When you can cultivate the opening of your own heart, you embrace the eagle vision. Eagle then brings the message to the Universe. What is the message you have for the eagle?"*

Vinyasa to Plank

Vasisthasana Prep – weave theme: *"Sometimes the way we take a stand has to change. When you feel the weight of the world on your shoulders, find a way to release it. Harness the energy you create with an open heart and rise up to the challenge of balancing on your hand."*

Tadasana

Vrksasana

Utthita Hasta Padangustasana – teach to open and set the hip and prep for Vasisthasana

Adho Mukha Svanasana – teach form, set shoulders and transition into Vasisthasana

Brigid's Cross

Parivrtta Upavistha Konasana

Upavistha Konasana

Janu Sirsasana

Setu Bandha Sarvangasana

Urdhva Dhanurasana – 3 rounds

Apanasana

Savasana

The Closing: * *"This is the Age of Empowerment. This is when we learn to claim our power, stop handing it over to others and release the chains that have kept us small or hidden. It is time to claim your true identity. Once you are at peace with your self, then you will be able to anchor and create the energy for the new world. Join the masses! Take a Stand!"*

Lila: The Playful Dance of Creation

This is a class that links movement with breath by using vinyasa to transition from one asana to the next.

The Opening: *"Lila is Sanskrit for playfulness. It's the play between the energies of Shiva and Shakti, purusha and prakruti. It is the playful dance of creation. Purusha, the spirit or soul, never changes. Much like the asanas, the general look or form never changes. But if we are able to invoke lila or playfulness, then the power of prakruti (creative nature) in the material world in all of us brings forth subtle changes in the soul. Let this playfulness be your inspiration in class and off the mat as we create this new way of living together in lila."*

Tadasana then Uttanasana – allow for movement, sway back and forth. Keep the hips square over the ankles and just move the upper body. The legs represent purusha, the form that never changes. The torso is prakruti, the creation of something new.

Adho Mukha Svanasana – the torso remains still, the legs move – press out the heels, sway the hips but keep a firm foundation in the hands. Playful jump into Uttanasana. Uttanasana changes into Parsva Uttanasana – again teaching that the form of the legs stays the same, upper body flexes to one side and then the other.

Adho Mukha Svanasana to Chaturanga Dandasana to Bhujangasana – teach shoulder openers. Change the form into Urdvha Mukha Svanasana – the arms stay the same, the legs move to create a new form.

Vinyasa to Salambasana – anchor the feet, pubic bone and play with lifting the heart on the inhalation and release down on the exhalation. Pause, then switch the breath: exhale to lift, inhale to lower.

Vinyasa to lunge – float fingers off the floor. Right hand reaches forward, left hand back. With each exhale, switch the arms. Do 4 rounds. Switch sides and do left hand forward, right hand back, exhale switch. Complete 4 rounds. Here, you can talk about the play in the arms while the soul (the legs) stay the same.

Vinyasa to lunge into lunge with a twist – playfully flow from lunge to lunge with a twist (4 rounds). Repeat on the other side.

Virabhadrasana II – have some fun here and go from reverse Virabhadrasana II (also called Sun Warrior) to Virabhadrasana II to Parsvakonasana. Back to Virabhadrasana II, reverse Virabhadrasana II, Virabhadrasana II to Parsvakonasana. Do 4 rounds, connecting movement with breath. Keep the legs firmly planted as purusha. The upper body does the movement. Repeat on the other side.

Prasarita Paddattonasana into Parvritti Prasarita Paddattonasana. Hips stay square as you use the breath to go into and out of the twist. Switch sides.

Vasisthasana playful flow – from plank, revolve into Vasisthasana side plank version, back to plank, to the other side. Move with the breath. Here the legs and core are the focus of the soul, they stay the same as you transition and change the arms. Do 4 rounds of this playful flow.

Vinyasa to seated Upavistha Konasana to Parvrtti Upavistha Konasana playful flow. Ground the femur bones into the earth to create stability as you flow.

Hold Ardha Matsyendrasana I prep (closed twist) then transition into Ardha Matsyendrasana I (open twist). The legs stay the same, the torso twists. Repeat on the other side.

Dandasana to Paschimottanasana to Purvottanasana.

Supta Eka Hasta Padasana to Parivrtta Supta Padangusthasana 4 rounds.

Supta Balasana to Savasana

The Closing: *"Cultivate lila in your daily life. Notice that although circumstances around you may change, your soul essence, your true inherent nature remains the same. Sometimes we may feel lost in our surroundings. That is the energy of prakruti, the creative nature dancing with purusha, the never changing soul. Embrace the playful dance of the two."*

Seeing the World Upside Down: A Lesson in Darshana.

Here's a class theme I use to teach headstand. (Only teach headstand to students who have been practicing with you for more than a year. Teach only headstand prep to beginners). With each inversion, teach your students to see the world from another perspective.

The Opening: *"The Sanskrit word darshana means 'to see', 'sight', 'view'. Sometimes we have to hold up the mirror with which we can look inside to view one's self. Yoga means to come together, to unite, to join. We can come to join our spirit with our practice by directing our thoughts to our practice. Yoga allows us to obtain what we perceive as unattainable. Yoga is change. We yoke, or join our thoughts with the feelings in our bodies by directing our attention toward the activity that is our asana practice. As our thoughts fade, our yoga brings us closer to the Divine and we begin to feel in harmony with a higher power; we can act kinder and be more attentive. Where do we start? How do we do this? By removing the obstacles in our way. How do we remove the obstacles? By seeing the world upside down."*

Uttanasana

Adho Mukha Svanasana – look behind you to see upside down

Wide legged Uttanasana – get another view of the world this way

Vinyasa to Bhujangasana – open your heart

Adho Mukha Svanasana to Dolphin

Pincha Mariyasana

Tadasana – teach alignment of shoulders

Virabhadrasana I into Baddha Hasta Parsvakonasana – different view

Adho Mukha Svanasana

Parivrtta Adho Mukha Svanasana – different view

Sirsasana Prep

Sirsasana

Balasana to Parivrtta Balasana

Ardha Matseyendrasana I prep

Ardha Matseyendrasana I

Janu Sirsasana – wide and bow through legs

Parivrtta Janu Sirsasana

Janu Sirsasana

Windshield Wipers

Setu Bandha Sarvangasana – 3 rounds

Savasana

The Closing: *"We can begin to practice being whole. We must incorporate all aspects of the self, step by step just as we did in our asana practice today. We must include being whole even in relationships with others, in our own behaviors, our health, our breathing and our meditation. Yoga makes us whole. The root of the word whole is holy. Holy means to heal. Join together in yoga and heal your soul by seeing the world upside down."*

Take a Look at Yourself – Make a Change

Sometimes you can get themes from music. I found inspiration in the lyrics of Michael Jackson's song *Man in the Mirror*. This class is all about creating change in asana, by building upon a strong foundation. I taught that the soul remains the same through every incarnation. It's the body and experiences that change in order for you to learn. I then encourage the students to create subtle changes in each pose and in their bodies.

The Opening: *"Reflect on the past year. Have you created any change in your life or are you still trotting along, doing the same old thing. In a world that is constantly changing, what have you done to keep up? Are you lagging behind? How have you evolved to help create change in both your life and in your practice or even in the world? In our practice today, we will learn how to keep a solid foundation in order to feel supported as we change. Your soul remains the same in every incarnation. It's your body and experiences that change. Let's learn how to translate this change into our practice."*

Table – change into variation with opposite arm and leg extending forward. Change that by extending the same arm and leg out toward the right and left side of the room. Use a lot of core strength, shoulder alignment, and balanced action to stay stable in this sequence. You will allow a rest period in Balasana after the three changes have occurred.

Adho Mukha Svanasana – set a solid foundation. Teach alignment. Change into three-legged dog with an open hip. Change by encouraging a bigger opening in the hip, let the leg that's lifted step down to the floor changing three-legged dog into flip the dog and into Wild Thing.

Rest in Balasana

Step into lunge. Lunge changes into a floating lunge which changes into lunge with a twist, hands in anjali mudra, then they can be encouraged to touch the floor either inside the front foot or outside (which is a more challenging version). Transition back to Uttanasana to release the back.

Warrior 2 changes into Reverse Sun Warrior, create a solid foundation and reiterate how the legs maintain stability, like the soul. The legs don't change, just the upper body does.

Change back into Warrior 2 and then Extended Side Angle with the front arm resting on the knee. Sense the weight on the front leg and create change (balanced action) by activating the back inner thigh more to make the front elbow feel lighter. Encourage a deeper, wider stance, as they did in lunge in order to teach change by going deeper and perhaps releasing the front arm to the floor outside the foot (Parsvakonasana). Change back into elbow on knee version and transition out to Uttanasana.

Tree Pose changes in the arms. Set a solid foundation in the legs, hug the midline and hold hands in anjali mudra at the heart. Create a distraction and change the arms by passing hands in front of face, then extend up, interlace last three fingers, cross the thumbs. Change by opening the arms out to the side. On the second side, create change by encouraging that they interlace fingers and cross their thumbs the non-dominate way.

Dandasana changes into a small back bend then changes into Purvottanasana.

Janu Sirsasana starts with the foot resembling Tree Pose then changes into a wider leg version and then changes into a twisting version.

Knee-to-Chest changes into the knee pulling up closer to the shoulder then it changes into Half Happy Baby. Other side does the sequence then the whole thing changes into Full Happy Baby.

Savasana can change by using props for support.

The Closing: *"Start to make little changes in your life. Begin by looking at yourself in the mirror and contemplate the question, 'Am I ready to change my ways?' In the words of the late Michael Jackson, 'If you want to make the world a better place, take a look at yourself and make that change.' "*

Sanskrit Used in Chapter Sixteen

Parvatasana – mountain pose, palms up

Vasisthasana – sage Vasistha's pose

Vrksasana – tree pose

Utthita Hasta Padangustasana – extended hand to big toe pose

Lila – playfulness

Shiva – auspicious one, the destroyer, part of the tri-murti

Shakti – cosmic energy

Purusha – the witness to creation

Prakruti – creative nature

Salambasana – locust pose

Ardha Matsyendrasana – half lord of the fish pose

Supta Eka Hasta Padasana – reclined hand to foot pose (half happy baby pose)

Parivrtta Supta Padangusthasana – revolved hand to big toe pose

Darshana – to see, sight, view

Pincha Mariyasana – peacock pose

Parivrtta Adho Mukha Svanasana – revolved downward facing dog pose

Sirsasana Prep – headstand prep pose

Sirsasana – headstand

Parivrtta Balasana – revolved child's pose

Parivrtta Janu Sirsasana – revolved head of the knee pose

Anjali mudra – a gesture of gratitude holding palms together and thumbs press gently against the heart center

Build Your Sequence Template

Quick Reference Template:

The Opening

Seated Centering

Warm Up

Heat Building Sequence

Standing Asana

Balance Asana

Seated Twisting Asana

Seated Asana

Cool Down

Inversions (Setu Bandha Sarvangasana for beginners)

The Closing

Relaxation: Savasana

The Opening:

Seated Centering:

Warm Up: facilitate movements in the big joints, big muscles first (3-4 asanas)

Heat building sequence: can be in the form of Surya Namaskar (4 rounds) or standing asana (4 asanas)

Standing Asana: teach the form, weave the theme (4-5 asanas)

Balance Asana: standing (1-2 asanas)

Seated Twisting Asana: (1 asana)

Seated Asana: (1-2 asanas)

Cool Down: forward folds (2-3 asanas)

Inversions: (Setu Bandha Sarvangasana, for beginners)

The Closing:

Relaxation: Savasana

Build Your Sequence Template

Quick Reference Template:

The Opening

Seated Centering

Warm Up

Heat Building Sequence

Standing Asana

Balance Asana

Seated Twisting Asana

Seated Asana

Cool Down

Inversions (Setu Bandha Sarvangasana for beginners)

The Closing

Relaxation: Savasana

The Opening:

Seated Centering:

Warm Up: facilitate movements in the big joints, big muscles first (3-4 asanas)

Heat building sequence: can be in the form of Surya Namaskar (4 rounds) or standing asana (4 asanas)

Standing Asana: teach the form, weave the theme (4-5 asanas)

Balance Asana: standing (1-2 asanas)

Seated Twisting Asana: (1 asana)

Seated Asana: (1-2 asanas)

Cool Down: forward folds (2-3 asanas)

Inversions: (Setu Bandha Sarvangasana, for beginners)

The Closing:

Relaxation: Savasana

Build Your Sequence Template

Quick Reference Template:

The Opening
Seated Centering
Warm Up
Heat Building Sequence
Standing Asana
Balance Asana
Seated Twisting Asana
Seated Asana
Cool Down
Inversions (Setu Bandha Sarvangasana for beginners)
The Closing
Relaxation: Savasana

The Opening:

Seated Centering:

Warm Up: facilitate movements in the big joints, big muscles first (3-4 asanas)

Heat building sequence: can be in the form of Surya Namaskar (4 rounds) or standing asana (4 asanas)

Standing Asana: teach the form, weave the theme (4-5 asanas)

Balance Asana: standing (1-2 asanas)

Seated Twisting Asana: (1 asana)

Seated Asana: (1-2 asanas)

Cool Down: forward folds (2-3 asanas)

Inversions: (Setu Bandha Sarvangasana, for beginners)

The Closing:

Relaxation: Savasana

Build Your Sequence Template

Quick Reference Template:

The Opening
Seated Centering
Warm Up
Heat Building Sequence
Standing Asana
Balance Asana
Seated Twisting Asana
Seated Asana
Cool Down
Inversions (Setu Bandha Sarvangasana for beginners)
The Closing
Relaxation: Savasana

The Opening:

Seated Centering:

Warm Up: facilitate movements in the big joints, big muscles first (3-4 asanas)

Heat building sequence: can be in the form of Surya Namaskar (4 rounds) or standing asana (4 asanas)

Standing Asana: teach the form, weave the theme (4-5 asanas)

Balance Asana: standing (1-2 asanas)

Seated Twisting Asana: (1 asana)

Seated Asana: (1-2 asanas)

Cool Down: forward folds (2-3 asanas)

Inversions: (Setu Bandha Sarvangasana, for beginners)

The Closing:

Relaxation: Savasana

Build Your Sequence Template

Quick Reference Template:

The Opening
Seated Centering
Warm Up
Heat Building Sequence
Standing Asana
Balance Asana
Seated Twisting Asana
Seated Asana
Cool Down
Inversions (Setu Bandha Sarvangasana for beginners)
The Closing
Relaxation: Savasana

The Opening:

Seated Centering:

Warm Up: facilitate movements in the big joints, big muscles first (3-4 asanas)

Heat building sequence: can be in the form of Surya Namaskar (4 rounds) or standing asana (4 asanas)

Standing Asana: teach the form, weave the theme (4-5 asanas)

Balance Asana: standing (1-2 asanas)

Seated Twisting Asana: (1 asana)

Seated Asana: (1-2 asanas)

Cool Down: forward folds (2-3 asanas)

Inversions: (Setu Bandha Sarvangasana, for beginners)

The Closing:

Relaxation: Savasana

Notes

Shine Your Light – Make Hearts Sing

"People are like stained-glass windows. They sparkle and shine when the sun is out, but when the darkness sets in their true beauty is revealed only if there is light from within."
~ Elisabeth Kübler-Ross

Allow your themes to send out positive messages of love and light. It begins with shining the light in your own heart.

May you continue to bring happiness to the masses
May you continue to shine your light for others to follow
May you continue to create themes in your yoga classes that bring about this shift in consciousness
May you continue to be that catalyst for change
May you continue to make your own heart sing

My intention is to always and all ways teach that I do not have the answers, that you have your own. I am merely the facilitator here to guide you on your journey.

With love and light,
Noelle Cormier

Lightning Source UK Ltd.
Milton Keynes UK
UKOW01f1401291016
286317UK00029B/149/P